# PLAY BALL!
# THE OFFICIAL
# LITTLE LEAGUE®
# FITNESS GUIDE

Other books by Champion Press

*30 Exercises for Better Golf*

*Shoulder and Arm Exercises for Baseball Players*

*Ejercicios de Hombro y del Brazo para
Jugadores de Béisbol*

# PLAY BALL!
## THE OFFICIAL
## LITTLE LEAGUE®
## FITNESS GUIDE

**FRANK W. JOBE, M.D.**

**TEAM PHYSICIAN
LOS ANGELES DODGERS
AND**

**ASSOCIATE CLINICAL PROFESSOR OF SURGERY
(ORTHOPAEDICS)
UNIVERSITY OF SOUTHERN CALIFORNIA**

**DIANE RADOVICH MOYNES, M.S., R.P.T.**

**ASSISTANT ADMINISTRATOR
CENTINELA HOSPITAL MEDICAL CENTER**

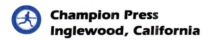

**Champion Press
Inglewood, California**

Published by Champion Press
Centinela Hospital Medical Center
555 East Hardy Street
Inglewood, California 90307

Champion Press is a registered trademark of
Centinela Hospital Medical Center

Production Coordination: Michael Bass & Associates
Cover: Archie Boston Design
Text Design: Nancy Benedict
Illustrations: Rik Olson
Cover Illustrator: Sid Bingham

Manufactured in the United States of America

Library of Congress Cataloging-in-Publication Data

Jobe, Frank W.
  Play ball!

  Rev. ed. of: The official Little League fitness guide / Frank W. Jobe, Diane Radovich Moynes. c1984.
  Includes index.
  1. Baseball for children — Training. 2. Physical fitness for children. 3. Little League Baseball, inc. 4. Exercise for children. I. Moynes, Diane Radovich. II. Jobe, Frank W. Official Little League fitness guide. III. Little League Baseball, inc. IV. Title.
GV875.6.J63   1986   796.357'62   86-17402
ISBN 0-936691-01-8

# ACKNOWLEDGEMENTS

We've enjoyed writing this, but books like this don't get written without lots of help. Some of the people who made important contributions are listed below.

Creighton Hale, Ph.D., President of the Little League, has offered valuable counsel and support throughout.

Russ Stromberg, President of Centinela Hospital, and Ann McClanathan, Vice President, have been unwavering in their enthusiasm and support of the project.

Eric Tuckman, Centinela's Legal Counsel, made pertinent comments and provided useful background information.

Dr. Ian Kramer of the Centinela Hospital Emergency Room reviewed our first-aid material and made sure we were up-to-date on all procedures.

Mary Bing, R.D., nutritional consultant to the Los Angeles Dodgers, is responsible for the sample menu section and review of the food section.

Jeff Mason, who does a great job coaching in the Chandler, Arizona, school system, shared his warm-up routines for infielders and outfielders.

## ACKNOWLEDGMENTS

Many of the exercises for strengthening and flexibility were adapted from the programs Clive Brewster, M.S., R.P.T., developed for his patients at the Kerlan-Jobe Orthopaedic Clinic.

The original manuscript went through a lot of changes, all of which were typed by Janice White.*

F.W.J.
D.R.M.

*Assistance for the second edition was provided by Nancy Sidon and Jeanne Bertolli.

# FOREWORD

Centinela Hospital Medical Center is a sports medicine
center where athletes come for treatment. Doctors here
take care of the professional baseball, football, hockey and
basketball teams. They also work with individual athletes
in all sports from around the country and throughout the
world.

The Biomechanics Laboratory at the hospital uses
computers, cameras and other equipment to understand
body movement in sports. Research here has helped us
pick the best exercises for baseball players. Other studies
look at golf, swimming and tennis. But, we don't only look
at sports. We also help kids and grown-ups who have
trouble walking or climbing stairs.

Meanwhile, our baseball research goes on. We are
now working on the big muscles of the back. We have
already learned a lot about the shoulder: how it gets hurt,
how to keep it from hurting and how to make it work
better after an injury. We understand better what happens
when you throw a curveball, and think that probably the

total number of pitches in games and practices is more important than what kind of pitch you throw.

To pick the best exercises for baseball players, we had to look at professionals. These athletes came to the Laboratory and we put special equipment on them to "hear" what each muscle says. We also took high-speed pictures, so that every motion—even the tiniest move—could be seen.

Once all the equipment was ready, each player warmed up and threw until he was comfortable. Then we turned on the lights and the cameras and gave the "go" signal. Cameras took pictures from overhead, in front, and on the side. Later on, we looked at each film frame and linked it to the muscle information. In this way, we studied shoulder muscles, back muscles and upper and lower arm muscles. All of this was put together with other things we know about general conditioning, food, and first aid to make a complete program for Little League.

# CONTENTS

# NOTE TO KIDS, PARENTS, AND COACHES

Fun should be the most important thing everyone gets from playing baseball. No one is perfect and everyone makes mistakes. Of course, it is disappointing to play and not win. Winning *is* fun, but just playing and knowing you played your best also count. Keeping in shape will make you feel better and perform better. Playing baseball, paying attention to how you throw and run and hit, will help you improve both coordination and physical skills.

Playing as part of a team is fun, and the experience will probably benefit you throughout your life. The friends you make are important, too. One of the nicest things about Little League is that you meet and get to know lots of different people—other kids on your team, kids on other teams, and your coaches. Little League was founded by people who understood that enjoying the game, learning to work with friends, and developing physical skills should all be essential parts of everyone's experience.

If you are a parent, coach, or friend of a Little League player, you also need to keep this in mind: a Little Leaguer can see if you react to the game with anxiety, anger, or frustration, either consciously or unconsciously. He or she needs to know that family and friends support the concepts of good sportsmanship and fun on which Little League is based.

To keep having fun, though, it is necessary to keep healthy and fit. This book should help with that. It was written by the doctors and physical therapists at Centinela Hospital in Inglewood, California, where the Dodgers and Angels and many other major-league ballplayers go to be tested and treated for injuries.

The book is divided into chapters that suggest ways to get into shape for playing. The first chapter has some thoughts about how to avoid getting hurt. The next chapter discusses conditioning. The third chapter shows good ways to warm up and stretch. After that, if an injury does occur, the next chapter tells you what to do in an emergency. The last chapter talks about eating right to play your best.

Putting all this together will help make your Little League experience a good one. Remember, though, that just because we've said it here, you needn't follow everything *exactly.* There are many ways of doing things, and we certainly haven't covered them all. The general principles of conditioning, warm-up, and flexibility are the important parts. By following these, you can play your best while decreasing the risk of hurting yourself.

# PLAY BALL!
# THE OFFICIAL
# LITTLE LEAGUE® 
# FITNESS GUIDE

# CHAPTER ONE

# Preventing Injuries

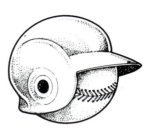

The old saying that an ounce of prevention is worth a pound of cure is true about athletic injuries, too. One of the main reasons to spend some of your time before a game or practice doing warm-up and conditioning activities is that they will help you avoid injuries while you play. By staying in good condition, you can play your best for longer lengths of time. If your body is warmed up, your muscles are more limber, and this helps you to play better. When you're warmed up, you also have less chance of getting a painful injury, such as a muscle tear or ligament sprain. A player who does not stay in shape and warm up (including stretching) before a game or practice session is much more likely to get hurt.

There are a number of other things you and your teammates can do to prevent an injury. If you are a pitcher, wearing a warm-up jacket helps keep your shoulders warm and loose. During a practice session, you should start throwing easily. Then you can begin to pitch a little harder. However, you should never throw as hard as you can during practice. (Even in a game you should throw your hardest only once in a while.) So warm up before and warm down (or cool down) after each game or practice session, and try to have a regular conditioning program as well.

A special word about pitching: it is necessary to set a limit on the number of pitches that you throw during the week. The muscles, ligaments, and especially the bones in your shoulders and elbows are still growing. Pitching is a strenuous activity that puts repeated stress on all of these developing parts inside your arm. When you repeatedly throw the ball hard, damage can occur. That's why Little League recommends that you pitch no more than the equivalent of six innings each week. Though the pitching you do during games may seem like the only pitching that really counts, it isn't. Your shoulder and arm work just as hard during team practices and even when you are throwing at home. So, be sure that you keep track of your pitches during practices and games as well as the throwing you do at home with family and friends. You shouldn't become careless just because you're not playing in an "official" game: most sports doctors believe that the majority of injuries occur in pick-up and practice games at home, after the league games.

In the professional leagues, the most successful pitchers concentrate on throwing for accuracy, and this is just as important for Little League pitchers. Learning to pitch the ball right over the plate will be more worthwhile than working on other types of pitches such as curves and sliders. Your most effective pitch will probably be a well-placed fastball, and, after you warm up and do your exercises, it is the pitch least likely to hurt your arm. Curve balls have been accused of causing lots of arm trouble, especially elbow trouble, in the past. But as we learn more and more about pitching, it seems that general overuse is a bigger factor in elbow problems than is throwing a particular pitch. The curve ball itself probably isn't as "bad" as originally thought, but you're better off pitching for accuracy. We really don't know enough to say how many would be too many curve balls. It's a good idea, just on general principle, not to throw very many anyway. There is one pitch, however, that probably should not be thrown at this stage, and that is the slider. The technique for throwing a slider requires you to "snap" your elbow. Repeating that motion many times can break off chips of bone.

Sliding into a base to beat the tag is exciting, fun, and often good strategy. But some recent research shows that a number of players who slide into base head first injure a shoulder. What happens is that they jam their hand into the bag and this pushes the arm hard up into the socket. Problems occur when the force is so great that it makes the arm go partially or completely out of joint momentarily. If this happens, you should see a doctor who knows about shoulder problems in sports. Always slide in feet first.

Proper equipment also prevents injury. Go through a checklist each time you take the field:

■ *Helmet:* Is your helmet on? Is it one that fits? A helmet that is too big will fall off when you run or when you hit the ground to get out of the way of a wild pitch. And that may be the time when you need the helmet the most. A helmet that is too small will be difficult to put on and remove, and because it is uncomfortable, it will distract you from your game.

■ *Bat:* Select a bat that is the right length and weight for your body and skill. A bat that feels comfortable in your hands and one that you can swing fairly easily is best. A bat that is too long or too heavy will not only make you swing awkwardly and cut down on the number of hits you get, but it can also lead to an injury. Never throw the bat around after hitting or during a practice session.

■ *Shoes:* Everyone knows that it is important to wear the proper shoes for your sport. However, having well-fitted baseball shoes doesn't help if the shoelaces have become untied and you trip on the way to first. You may then miss the fun of getting on base and helping your team. But, more importantly, you can be injured and then not be able to play your best. And even if you can run with your shoes like that, shoes that aren't tied properly slow you down—you just can't run as fast and you may not beat that tag at second! By the way, metal cleats are not permitted in Little League, so make sure your shoes have either plastic or rubber cleats.

New shoes take time to "break in." Start out by wearing them for the first fifteen minutes of practice and then switch back to your old shoes. After a week or so on this schedule, your new shoes should feel good and not give you blisters. Two pairs of socks can help prevent blisters, too.

■ *Clothing:* The regular baseball uniform that you use for games should be comfortable enough to allow you to run, hit, and throw without any problems. The same is true for your practice clothes. Clothes that are too long or too big will get in your way; clothes that are too tight will keep you from moving well in all directions. A good time to tell if your clothes are too tight is during your stretching exercises. If you cannot stretch properly because your clothes fit too closely, then chances are you'll be uncomfortable during a practice or game. Clothes that are too loose can get in the way of your arm motions and cause you to strike out or make a bad throw.

# CHAPTER TWO

# Conditioning

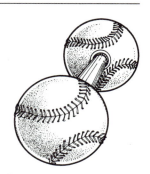

All athletes spend a lot of time getting into shape and staying in shape during their playing season. Good athletes make this a part of their everyday lives all year long. This getting into and staying in shape is known as *conditioning*. There are two kinds of conditioning: one has to do with being strong and limber, and the other determines how long you can exercise or play without getting tired.

The first type of conditioning should include exercises to strengthen not only your shoulders and arms but also your legs and trunk. Although it may not seem to take a great deal of strength to throw, hit, or catch a ball, doing these things well, over and over, requires both strength and coordination. The stronger you are, the farther you will be able to hit and throw.

Coordination is important, too. When ballplayers talk about "quickness," what they often mean is coordination. Being coordinated means that you can get your whole body—from your feet through your legs and trunk and up to your arms—to move smoothly. The better coordinated you are, the quicker you can get around to swing the bat, move in on a ground ball, or turn and throw out a base runner. One good way to become better coordinated is to repeat a certain movement over and over. That way the movement becomes automatic; your body does it almost without your mind having to think about it. This is what practice sessions are all about: practicing the pickoff throw from the pitcher to first base again and again, working on routine fly balls, and going over and over the relay from shortstop to second to first.

The exercises listed here are a good way to begin your conditioning program. Exercises should be done three times a week. Start the program by repeating the first exercise ten times without stopping, and continue through the rest of the group, doing each exercise the specified number of times. The whole group of exercises is called a *set.* When you can do one set of all these without becoming sore the next day, increase the number of repetitions by doing a second set. In the beginning, hold only a small amount of weight—such as one pound— and increase it very gradually as time goes on and you become stronger. Exercising three times a week is a good program. Remember to breathe normally as you exercise; don't hold your breath. To develop a "habit," we recommend exercising on Monday, Wednesday, and Friday. During the season, if strength gains have already been achieved, we recommend a "maintenance" program. If you play regularly, one day per week should do it. If you want to do more, then continue on the three-day program without making substantial increases in the weights. If you don't play regularly, work out on the strength program (exercise 1 to 12) at least two days per week.

You should not have to go out and buy a whole new set of weights to do these exercises. There are some weights you can buy, such as small barbells or sandbags. But you can use any number of other things for weights. You can make your own weight by putting sand or marbles into a heavy plastic bag and zipping or tying it shut. Or you may want to use a one-pound can in each hand or a tennis-ball can filled with sand. The important thing is to start. Use a light weight and increase it gradually.

Both boys and girls should be aware that when they lift weights in this way they are not going to develop large muscles. This will never occur in girls and will not take place in boys until they are older. However, baseball players should not build up big muscles like those of body builders. They do want to increase their strength, but improving coordination is most important. For this reason players should not concentrate on lifting a heavy weight once or twice but on lifting a lighter weight correctly many times, using the proper motion each time. Exercising in this way will promote both strength and coordination and will not damage any of the growing bones or muscles.

The second type of conditioning is designed to improve your body's energy delivery system. This delivery system is known as the *cardiovascular* system, and it also needs to be exercised, just as your muscles do. Just what is an energy delivery system? Well, it's the system that brings "food" to your muscles, and one of the main foods that muscles need is oxygen. Oxygen is found in the air we breathe, and exercising muscles must have a steady supply of it if they are going to function without getting tired. Your heart, lungs, and blood vessels are responsible for getting the necessary oxygen out of the air and delivered to the arm, leg, and trunk muscles that need it most while you are playing. If your cardiovascular system is in shape you can play ball without getting so tired in those late innings.

To get your cardiovascular system into shape you should begin what is called an *endurance training program*. There are many different exercises you can include in your training program, such as jogging, swimming, or bike riding. The important thing to remember about an endurance training program is that it is a strengthening program for your energy delivery system. This conditioning gets your heart and lungs into shape so that they can deliver oxygen to muscles more quickly and for longer periods of time. You can start by jogging for a short distance—maybe once or twice around the outside of the ball park. Do this three times a week. At first you are going to find that you feel out of breath or your legs are too tired to finish—maybe both. This means that your body isn't delivering enough oxygen to the muscles. Don't be discouraged; take a day off, then try jogging again. You'll notice that your heart beats faster while you're jogging and right afterward. This is good because it lets you know that your heart is being exercised. You'll also discover that jogging will get easier as you do it more and more. This is because your heart (which is really just a pump made of muscle) will get stronger and work better. To continue improving, slowly increase the number of times you jog around the park. A good schedule would be to add about a lap to your distance once every other week. For the first two weeks, try to run around the ball park twice on days you exercise. Every two weeks afterward, add one lap around the park (three times in the third week, four times in the fifth week, etc.).

The older you are and the heavier you are, the farther you should run. But don't do more than is fun. Pain isn't what you are after, conditioning is.

Let's talk for a minute about girls playing baseball. For a long time baseball was a sport for boys. Sometimes girls would play catch at home with their dads or brothers, but mostly they didn't play at all. Nowadays, with so much emphasis on fitness and physical activity, more and more girls are playing baseball. There isn't anything special about the way girls are built that keeps them from running and throwing as well as boys. Girls do tend to be just a little smaller and lighter than boys of the same age. However, whether you're a boy or a girl, practicing will develop your ability to run and throw well. That's why lifting weights, running, and practicing baseball skills are just as important for girls as for boys. Doing these things will not make girls big and muscular, nor will doing any of these athletic activities change or slow down the normal developmental process girls go through. And girls aren't likely to hurt themselves any more often or any differently than boys. Instead, exercising and playing baseball will help girls develop coordination and good muscle tone—important to them as well.

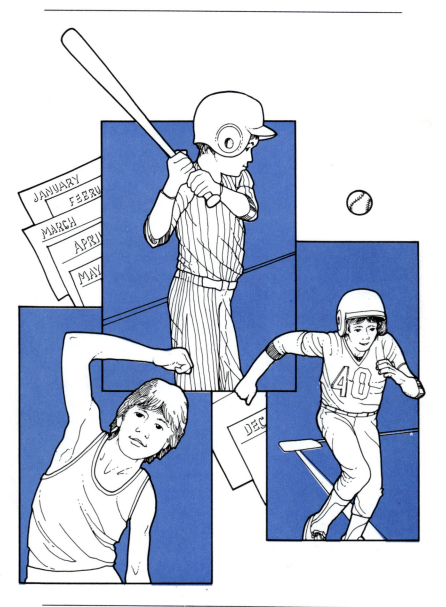

When it comes to conditioning for both boys and girls, remember the following:

■ Have a regular conditioning program that includes jogging or swimming or bicycling.

■ Keep up your conditioning all year round, not just right before and during baseball season.

■ You can exercise your arm, trunk, and leg muscles three times a week by doing the special strengthening exercises.

■ This is fun, not work. There should be no pain.

The first exercises are for your shoulder muscles. It's pretty easy to see why you need to have strong shoulder muscles for throwing and batting. Your ability to do these two important activities should be improved by these exercises. Next are exercises for the muscles further down your arm, followed by exercises for strengthening the thigh and calf muscles. Finally, there are two wrist exercises for athletes who want to do more.

# EXERCISE 1

## Shoulder Lifts

Stand or sit with your arms down at your sides. You can hold a small weight in each hand or use weights which tie around your wrist. Slowly lift your arms until they are straight out at your sides and then slowly lower them back down to your sides. Repeat this ten times. ■

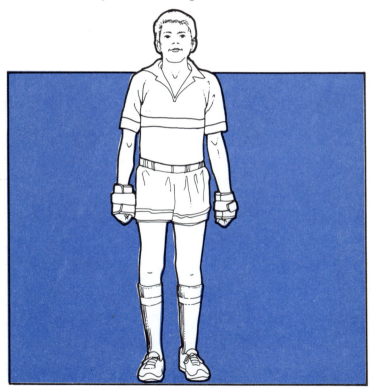

# Shoulder Lifts (cont.)

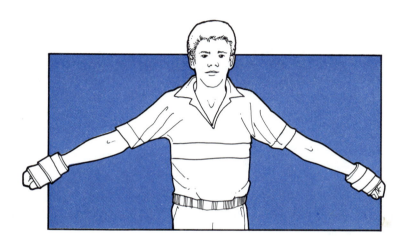

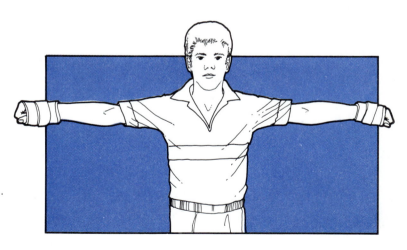

## EXERCISE 2

## Diagonal Shoulder Lifts

While standing or sitting, put your arms diagonally out from your shoulders. Turn your hands so that your thumbs are pointing down to the floor while you are holding the weights. Now raise your arms until they are shoulder high and then slowly lower them again. Repeat this ten times.

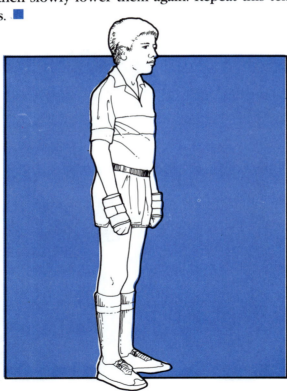

# Diagonal Shoulder Lifts (cont.)

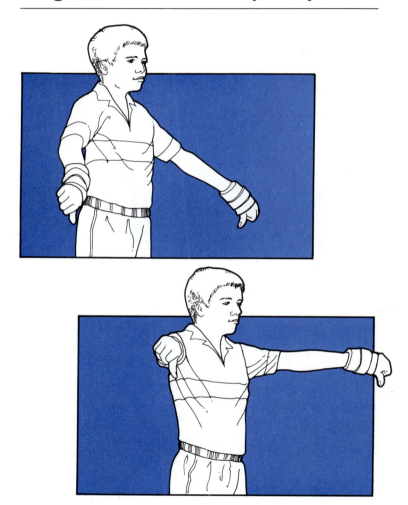

## EXERCISE 3

# Outward Shoulder Rotations

Lie on your side with your elbow close to your body. Slowly raise your hand, holding the weight, until it is pointing toward the ceiling, and then carefully lower it. Do ten repetitions. You should repeat this and the other arm exercises on the other side for good muscle balance. ◼

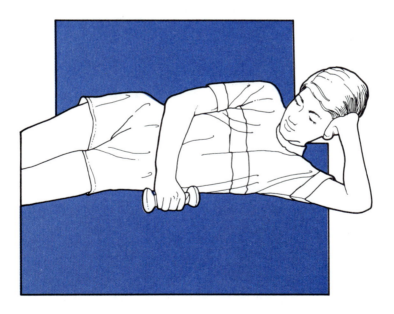

# Outward Shoulder Rotations (cont.)

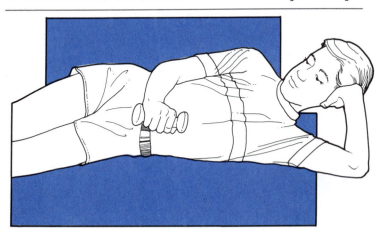

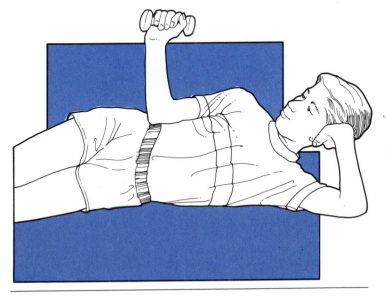

# EXERCISE 4

## Inward Shoulder Rotations

This time lie on your back. Again, hold your elbow close to your side. Move the hand holding the weight until it is pointing straight up. Return to the starting position and repeat ten times. Now repeat on the other side. ■

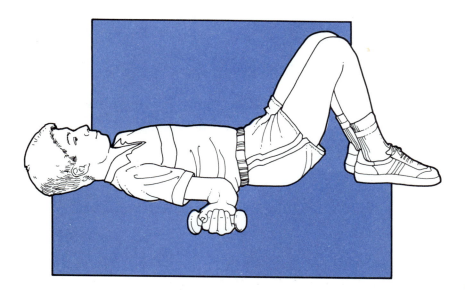

# Inward Shoulder Rotations (cont.)

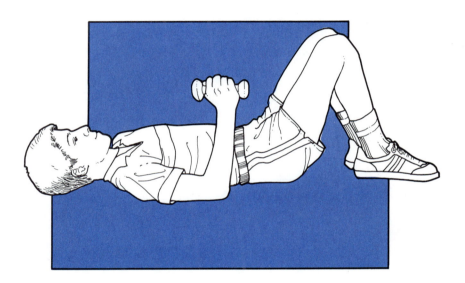

## EXERCISE 5

# Elbow Extensions

This is an exercise for the muscles further down your arm: While still on your back, place your hand on the floor above your shoulder, with your elbow pointing straight up. Raise your whole arm, holding the weight,

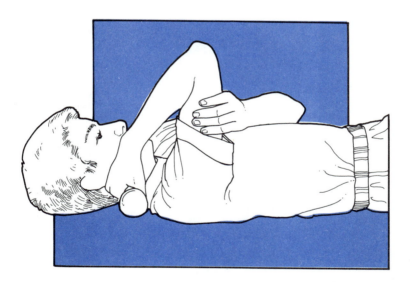

## Elbow Extensions (cont.)

until it is pointed toward the ceiling. Support the back of your arm with the other hand. Now slowly bend and straighten your elbow ten times. Then repeat with your other arm. ■

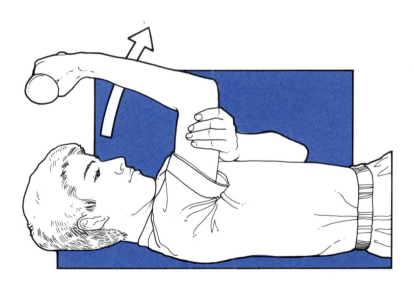

## EXERCISE 6

# Arm Curls

Here is another exercise for the muscles further down the arm: Sit or stand. Bend your arms at the elbow, your palms toward the ceiling. While holding the weight, slowly bend your elbow as far as it will go and then straighten it out again to the starting position. Repeat ten times on each side. ■

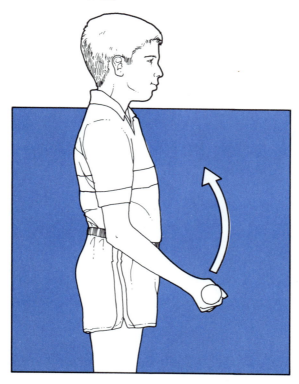

# Arm Curls (cont.)

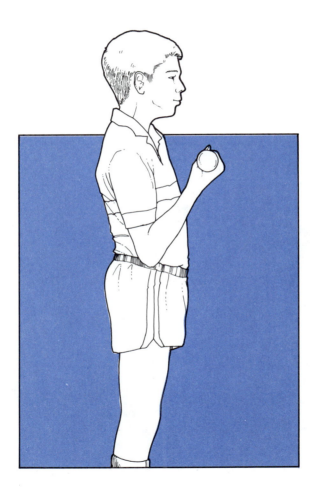

## EXERCISE 7

# Bent-knee Sit-ups

The trunk muscles are very important to ballplayers. Here is a good exercise for them: Lie on your back and bend your knees so that your feet are flat on the floor. Raise your head and trunk up until your hands can reach your knees, and then lie down again slowly. Do this exercise ten times as well. ■

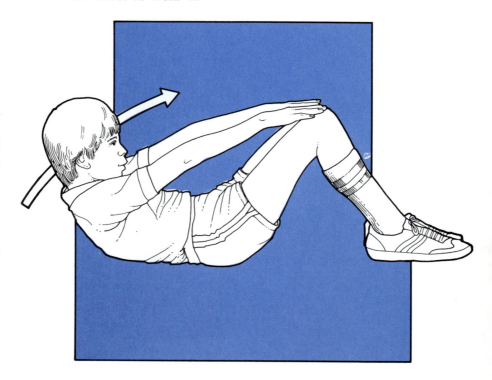

## EXERCISE 8

# Toe Raises

Don't forget the muscles further down your legs in your calves. Strengthen them by doing this exercise: Start with your feet flat on the ground and toes pointed straight ahead. Gradually go up on your toes as far as you can, then return to the foot-flat position. Repeat ten times. ■

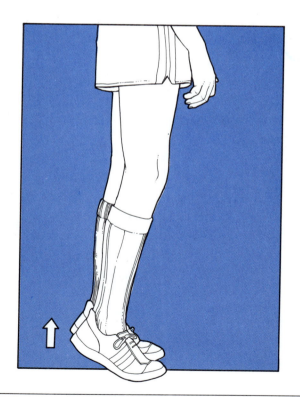

# EXERCISE 9

## Wall Push-ups

Stand next to a wall, with your feet about twelve inches out from the wall. Put your hands on the wall at shoulder level and lean in so that your face is close to the wall. Now, slowly push your body away until your arms are straight. This exercise is an easier version of a push-up done on the floor. It strengthens your arms and your shoulder blade muscles which are very important, especially to throwers. Repeat ten times. ■

# Wall Push-ups (cont.)

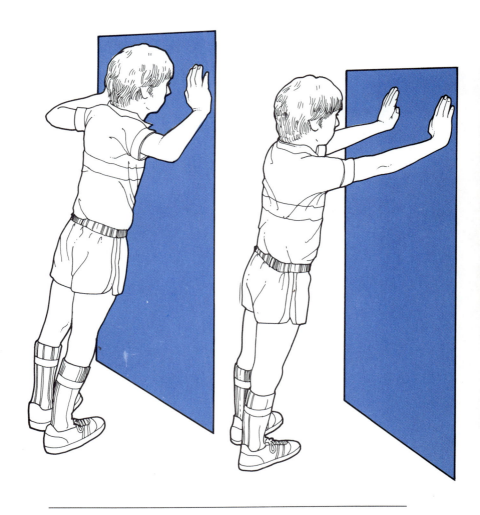

# EXERCISE 10

## Wall Slides

Strong leg muscles are necessary for all the running you do as a baseball player. Your thigh muscles can be strengthened by doing the following exercise: Lean backward against a wall with your feet about eight inches from the wall. Let yourself slide slowly down the wall until you are "sitting" on air. Hold this position and slowly count to five. Next, slide back to the standing position. Repeat five times. ■

## Wall Slides (cont.)

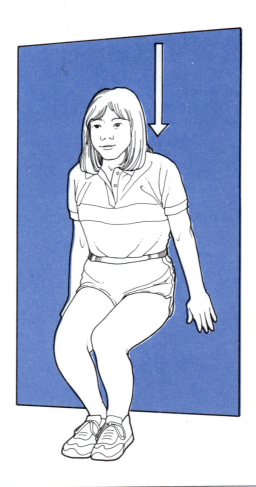

# EXERCISE 11

## Wrist Bends #1

If you want to do more, do this exercise for your wrists: Stand or sit with your arm bent at the elbow, your elbow close to your side. Hold a light weight or tennis-ball can filled with sand in your hand. Without moving your arm, bend your wrist slowly so that your palm is toward your chest. Slowly go back to the starting position and repeat 10 times. Now repeat on the other side. ◼

# Wrist Bends #1 (cont.)

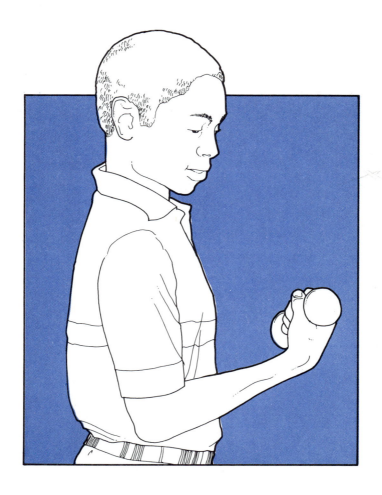

# EXERCISE 12

## Wrist Bends #2

Here is one more exercise for your wrists. Start from the same position shown in Exercise 11, but hold the weight so that your knuckles are toward the ceiling. Slowly bend your wrist toward your chest and return to the starting position. Do this ten times with one arm, then ten more with the other. ■

# Wrist Bends #2 (cont.)

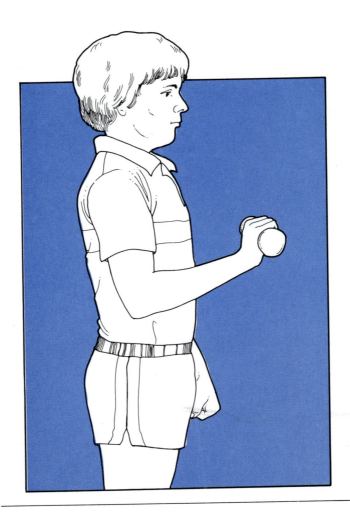

# CHAPTER THREE

# Warming Up & Stretching

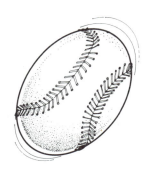

Warm-up is a routine to get both your mind and your whole body ready for the physical demands of playing baseball or any other sport. You should do your warm-up exercises right before you go out on the field. Warm-up is really a good name for these activities because they actually raise your body's temperature. Not only that, they usually increase your heart rate, blood pressure, and breathing rate. That's because during warm-up the amount of blood flowing to muscles increases to carry all the extra oxygen needed by the muscles during exercise. By getting your heart and other body parts ready before playing ball, you can reduce the wear and tear on these tissues when play begins. A very important effect of warm-up is that it makes your muscles more flexible; it limbers you up. Cold muscles are stiffer, and stiff muscles can be injured more easily. Warm muscles move more easily and react faster.

You may have heard commercials on television for creams you rub on your shoulder, arm, or leg to get warmed up. These products don't do anything that a hot shower can't do. The cream irritates your skin so that more blood comes to that area. It is kind of like warming up from the outside. What is really best is to warm up from the inside; that is, to get the muscles and ligaments themselves warmed up. Warmed-up skin won't help you play better or get going faster.

Warm-up exercises can be either general or specific. General warm-up exercises use many muscles to raise the temperature of your whole body. An example of a general warm-up would be a fast walk, a slow jog, or running in place. The effects of a general warm-up can last as long as thirty minutes. Specific warm-up exercises, on the other hand, are used to prepare only certain muscles for activity. Specific warm-ups do not use very many muscles, but each exercise will help get you ready for the exact requirements of your position.

Since you are a baseball player, your specific warm-up should also include swinging a bat and throwing a ball. Warming up the muscles in your arms is particularly important. Even if you've jogged around the park a few times and done exercises to get your body temperature up, that's not enough. You can injure yourself if you throw hard before your arm has been properly warmed up. Throw only at slow speed during warm-up; don't throw as hard as you can. Throwing harder does not make your muscles warm up faster, it just makes it more likely that you'll get hurt. Start out by just tossing the ball easily. After a few tosses, you can begin to throw just a bit harder. At no time during the warm-up should you be throwing as hard as you can.

If you are an outfielder, you may be called upon to make a long throw in to one of the infielders. This can happen, as you know, at any time and with little warning. If you haven't warmed up before going out onto the field, you won't be able to throw as far or as forcefully. Also, if you haven't warmed up, you run a higher risk of hurting your arm from a vigorous throw. So if you are an outfielder, you ought to include some long throws in your warm-up routine. If you're an infielder, you might include running forward and fielding the ball as well as running to each side and fielding the ball. If you're a catcher, you need to be especially sure that your legs are properly warmed up so that moving in and out of a crouch will be easy. And, of course, if you'll be pitching, you should warm up your throwing arm very carefully, taking care to begin by just tossing the ball back and forth a short distance. Only after that has been done for a few minutes should you back up and toss the ball a bit further. Again, do that for a few minutes and then throw the ball a little harder. If you are a pitcher, you need a carefully regulated program to protect your arm from injury. If you haven't conditioned and warmed up properly, and if you don't use good form while pitching, then you are more likely to hurt yourself. Of course, if you pitch too much or practice too much at home between games, your chances of serious injury are increased. Be sure you get several days' rest between games in which you pitch.

Limit the number of pitches you make during practice and make easier throws. On off-days, practice about fifteen minutes and throw at three-quarter speed. It is our opinion that throwing an occasional curve ball is not nearly as dangerous as is throwing too much.

Exercises to limber up your muscles and joints are called *flexibility exercises,* or stretching exercises. The purpose of the warm-up is to get your heart working harder and pumping more blood to your muscles. The flexibility exercises will stretch out your muscles to their best working length. These stretching exercises should be done during warm-up and repeated after each practice. Being flexible in the kind of movements required in your sport reduces the risk of injury. A baseball player needs good flexibility in his whole body: at the wrist, elbow, and shoulder for throwing, at the hip for fielding, in the trunk for hitting and throwing, and in the legs for running.

Stretching exercises will make you more flexible. "Bounce" stretching isn't the best way to stretch. (These are stretches in which you hold a position and give a few quick bounces at the end.) It's probably better to do a static or "holding" stretch like the ones illustrated here. If holding these positions is too painful, you do not have to get into the exact positions shown in the pictures. Just try to come as close to the illustrations as you can. Place yourself in each position just until you begin to feel a little pain, hold it for about fifteen to twenty seconds, and then relax. You are the best one to judge when you are stretching properly. Repeat each stretch two to three times.

The list of exercises below is a good starting routine and can get you into the good habit of making sure your muscles are "loose." As you get older and play harder, more detailed warm-up routines become important.

A good pregame program combines warm-up and flexibility routines. Try a program like this:

1. Jog for ten minutes.

2. Do a set of stretching exercises.

3. Do a set of warm-up exercises.
   (a) legs
   (b) trunk
   (c) arms

Now you're ready to play!

All workouts should be followed by a warming-down period, sometimes known as *cool-down*. Cool-down helps prevent soreness by allowing blood to continue circulating smoothly as you cool off. It is basically just the opposite of warm-up: this time you reduce the pace of your activity, throw easily, and swing the bat slowly. Take a slow jog or a slow walk around the field and repeat your stretching exercises. This routine will help reduce the tendency to get sore muscles, especially after a long workout or tough game. The soreness can come from an accumulation in the muscle of waste products from exercise. A period of relatively low-intensity (so-called "light") exercise will keep blood flowing through the muscles which have been working. This blood flow will help "wash away" the waste products. The easy nature of the warm-down or cooling-down activity will not stress tired muscles even further.

It is fun to warm up and stretch as a team. But if you then sit on the bench for a couple of innings, you should swing a bat and do a few arm circles, trunk circles, and a quick jog out to your position before you begin play. Remember, if it has been more than thirty minutes since you warmed up and stretched with your team at the start of the game, many of the good effects, such as loose muscles and better blood flow, have worn off. You need to be warmed up just before *you* play because warm-up is for *your* body.

Here are some important points to remember about warm-up:

■ The purpose of warm-up is to increase the body temperature, so sweating is a good indication of how well you have achieved this purpose.

■ Warm-up should include stretching exercises.

■ Warm-up is important in preventing muscle soreness and injury as well as improving athletic performance.

Some important things to remember regarding stretching are:

■ You should learn to stretch properly and not do it in a painful manner.

■ Everyone is different, and what your body can do is different from what others can do, so don't compete with someone else in your stretching.

■ Stretching should be done both before and after workouts.

■ Stretching should be done slowly, without sudden, jerky movements.

■ Stretching can help reduce the soreness and tightness which sometimes occur after a particularly hard workout.

The following exercises make a good warm-up program for most sports because they include both general and specific warm-ups. Exercises for all parts of the body are included. Do each one carefully; speed is not important. You will know you are getting warmed up if you begin to sweat a little before you finish all the exercises.

## EXERCISE 13

# Head and Neck Circles

Make a circle with your head, going around first in one direction five times. Then reverse and make five circles in the opposite direction. ■

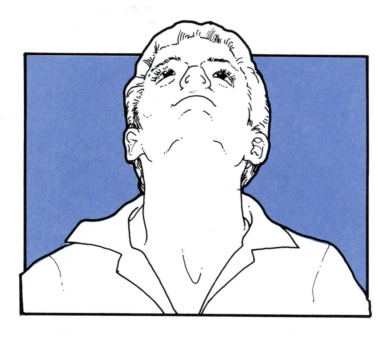

# Head and Neck Circles (cont.)

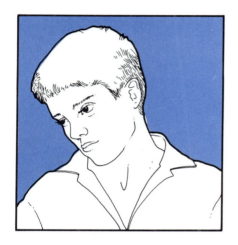

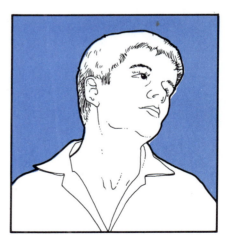

## EXERCISE 14

# Arm Circles

Hold your arms out to the side with the elbows straight.
Make five circles forward and five circles backward. ■

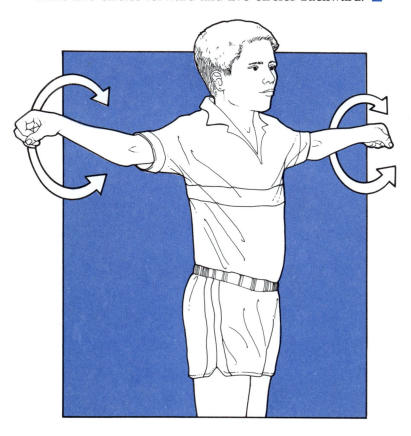

# EXERCISE 15

## Shoulder Shrugs

With your arms down at your sides, lift your shoulders toward your ears (in other words, just "shrug" your shoulders). Do this ten times. ■

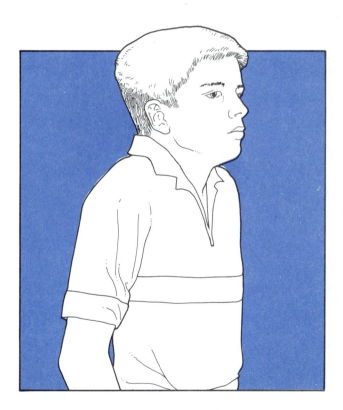

# EXERCISE 16

## Side Bends

While standing, bend to the right side and then stand up straight again. Do this five times and then five more times going to the left side. You can keep both hands on your hips or let one arm come overhead when you bend. ◼

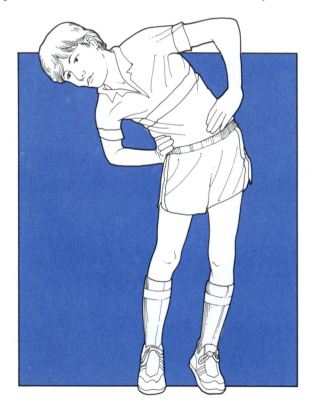

## Side Bends (cont.)

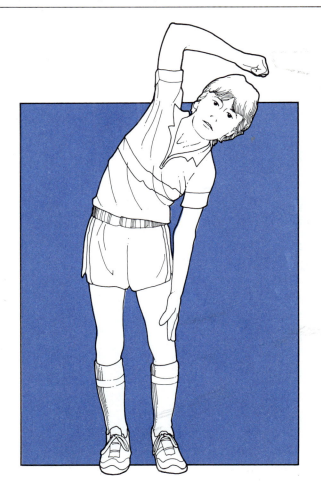

## EXERCISE 17

# Wrist and Hand Circles

Make five circles in each direction with your wrists and hands. ■

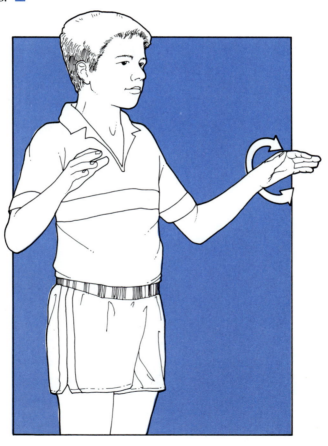

## EXERCISE 18

# Trunk Circles

Make a circle with your trunk, bending from the waist forward and around. Repeat five times. Then repeat five more times, circling in the other direction. ■

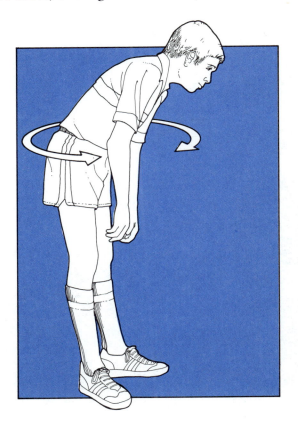

## EXERCISE 19

# Ankle Circles

Sit down on the ground and stretch your legs straight out in front of you. Make five circles inward with your feet and ankles, and then five circles outward. ■

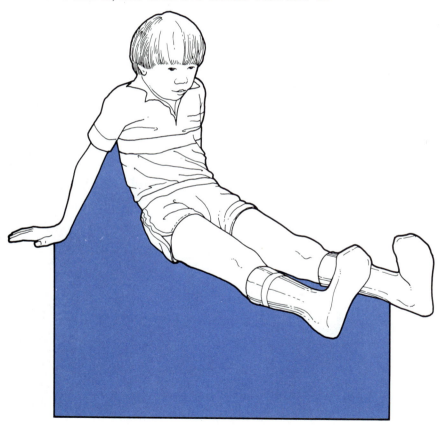

# Ankle Circles (cont.)

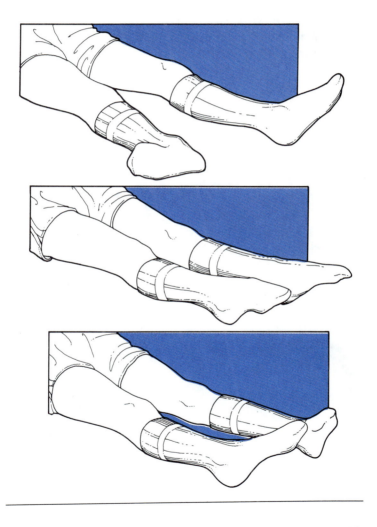

# EXERCISE 20

## Back Arches

While lying on your stomach, lift your head and legs up at the same time, arching your back. Lower them to the ground and repeat five times. ■

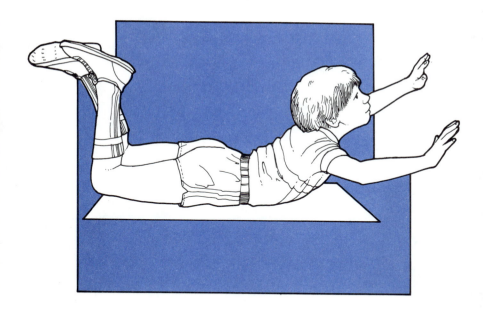

## EXERCISE 21

# *Running in Place*

Finally, stand up again and run in place. Count each step as one and keep going until you get to a hundred. ■

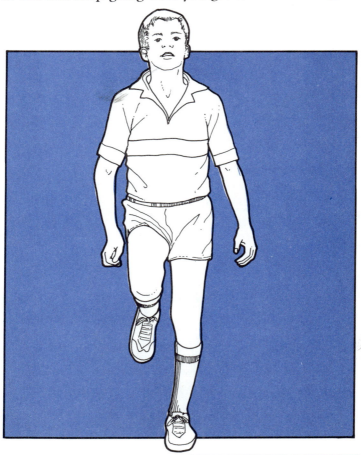

# EXERCISE 22

## Shoulder Stretches #1

Stand or sit, holding your throwing arm at the wrist with your other hand. Put your arm over your head and pull gently, feeling your upper arm against your head. You should feel the stretch inside your shoulder. ■

# Shoulder Stretches #1 (cont.)

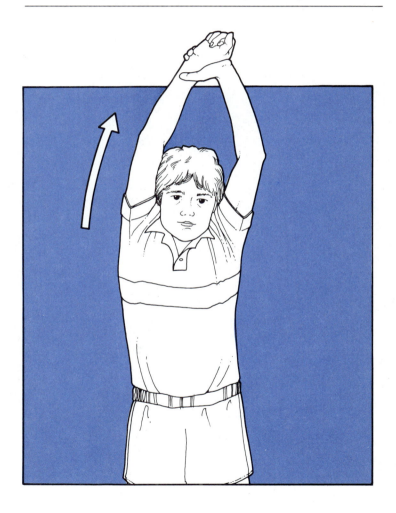

# EXERCISE 23

## Shoulder Stretches #2

Stand or sit, holding onto the elbow of your throwing arm with your other hand. Gently pull your throwing arm across your chest. You should feel the stretch inside your shoulder, especially at the back. ■

# Shoulder Stretches #2 (cont.)

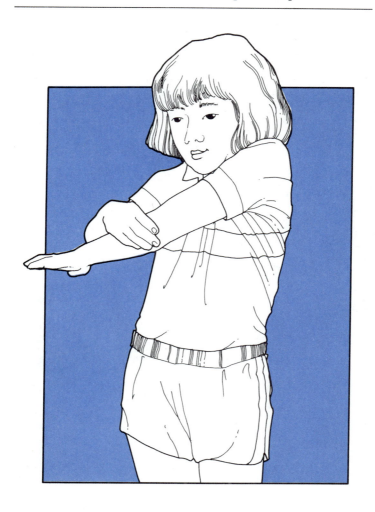

# EXERCISE 24

## Shoulder Stretches #3

Stand or sit with your pitching arm out to the side and your elbow bent. Move your arm back until you feel the stretch in the front of your shoulder. ■

# Shoulder Stretches #3 (cont.)

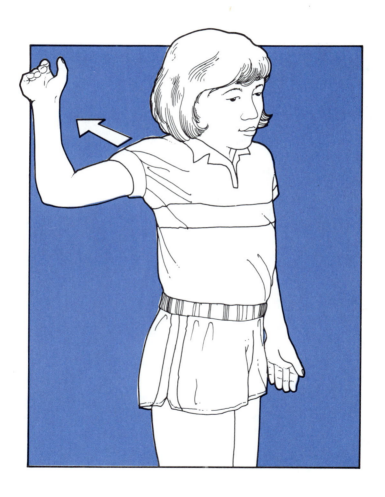

# EXERCISE 25

## Trunk Twisters

Stand or sit and twist your whole body all the way around to the right. Repeat, twisting all the way to the left. You should feel the stretch along your sides. ■

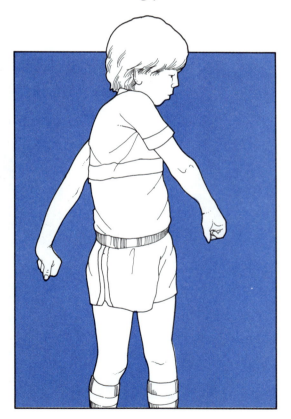

# Trunk Twisters (cont.)

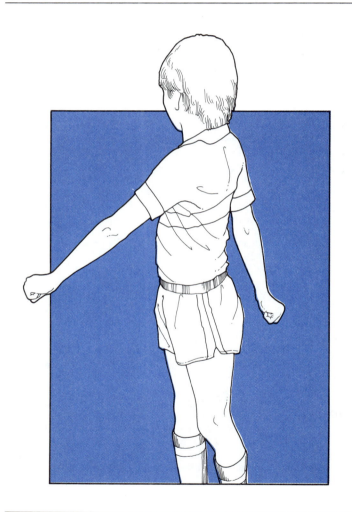

## EXERCISE 26

# Groin Stretches

Sit on the floor with your legs spread apart as far as possible. Lean forward as far as you can; keep your knees straight. You should feel the stretch along the inside of your thighs. ■

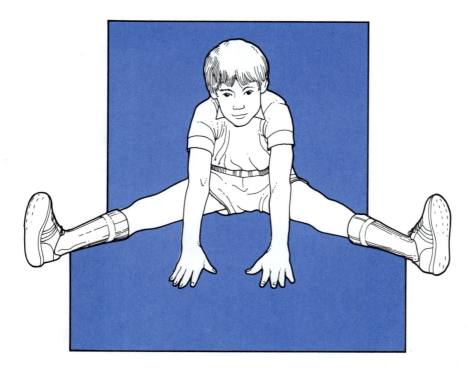

## EXERCISE 27

# Low Back Stretches

Lie on your back, bring one knee up, and pull the knee slowly toward your chest. Hold and repeat three times. Switch legs and repeat. ▪

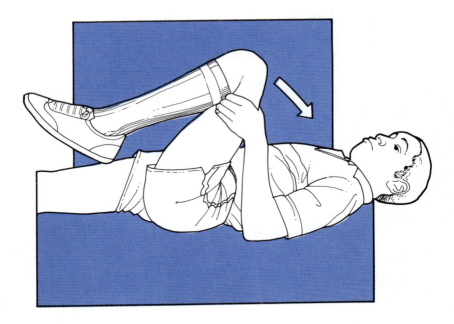

## EXERCISE 28

# Thigh Stretches #1

Sit on the floor. Stretch both legs out in front of you. Reach forward, touching your toes. Eventually, you want to lean forward far enough to put your head on your knees. You should feel the stretch along the backs of your legs. ∎

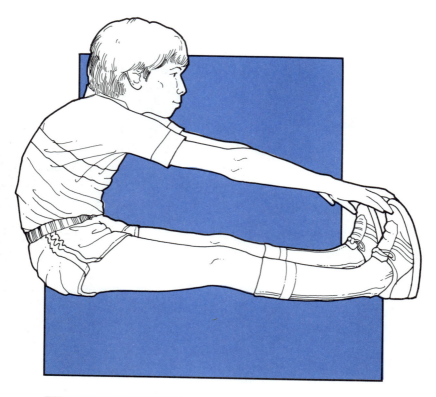

# Thigh Stretches #1 (cont.)

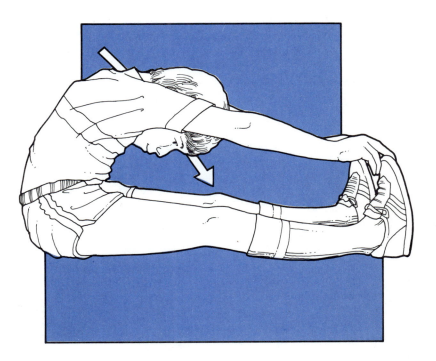

## EXERCISE 29

# Thigh Stretches #2

Sit on the floor with one leg stretched out in front of you. Bend the other knee and put your foot behind you. Lean backwards. You should feel the stretch along the front of your thigh. ■

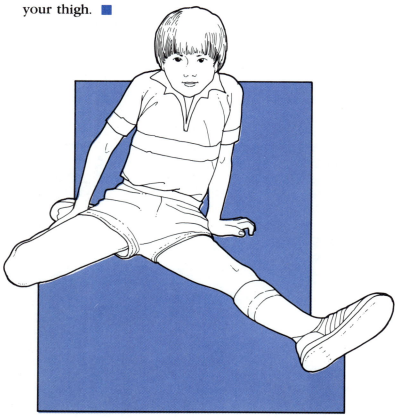

# EXERCISE 30

## Heel Cord Stretches

Lean up against a wall. Reach one leg behind you. Keep the knee straight, heel on the ground, and toes pointed forward. Slightly bend the leg that's closer to the wall. Lean forward. You should feel the stretch along the back of your calf. Repeat with the other leg. ■

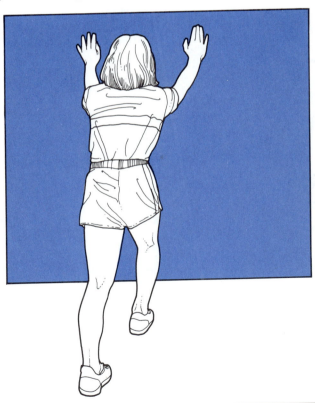

# CHAPTER FOUR

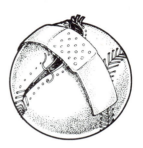

# In Case
# of Injury

Even if you are very careful, injuries and accidents can happen. Your team and your coach should be prepared for emergencies in several ways. Your coach should have a first-aid kit handy, equipped to treat cuts, blisters, bites, etc. The coach should know of a nearby doctor or a nearby hospital emergency room or urgent-care clinic that is available to treat injuries. The phone numbers of the doctor, the emergency room or clinic, and the local fire department or paramedic station should be on hand at all practices and games.

Some injuries, such as those that result in a sore elbow or painful shoulder, can occur over a long period of time. These injuries begin slowly and are often the result of repeated stress or overuse of muscles or bones that are not strong or limber enough to handle the force required. If you have these kinds of problems, then you may be pushing your body too hard or not warming up and stretching sufficiently. Pain is a sign that something is wrong: pay attention to what your body is telling you. Don't think that you have to "work through" the pain.

The best thing for an elbow or shoulder that is sore after a hard workout or game is rest. After a few days of rest, if the arm begins to hurt again when you play, you should tell your parents and go to a doctor who understands sports and sports injuries. Some cities have sports injury clinics that treat young athletes. Paying attention to pain at an early stage can help you prevent a more serious problem later. It is probably a *bad* idea to use ointments or creams that make a painful arm feel warm or tingly so it won't hurt and you can play. By using them, you are ignoring the message your body is sending about that shoulder or elbow.

Very few kids who play baseball develop elbow problems, and still fewer develop shoulder problems. However, if you throw too hard and too often you may develop a problem known as *Little League elbow.* This problem is due to an injury to the "growth center" in one of the bones of your arm. These growth centers are present in all the bones of your body, and they are exactly what their name seems to say: the place where growth occurs. It is possible to damage one of the growth centers in your arm if you ignore discomfort and attempt to "pitch through the pain." Most kinds of Little League elbow do not cause permanent damage, only discomfort while you are playing, and will get well with rest. There is one *rare* injury which usually comes on as you move from Little League to "Pony" League and which can be serious. Be wary about pitching with pain in the elbow.

Other kinds of injuries and accidents, like being hit

with a ball or breaking a bone, must be treated immediately. Here's what to do and what *NOT* to do:

**Bites and Stings**  Most insect bites and stings are not serious. Ice or coolant can help the itch or pain, and an antihistamine (such as in cold remedies) may help swelling and side effects such as itching. Additionally, pain relief can come from aspirin or an acetaminophen (such as Tylenol). The following insects are relatively dangerous: honeybees, black widow spiders (with hourglass-shaped red mark on bottom), brown recluse or "fiddleback" spiders, and scorpions. If a honeybee stings someone, the stinger and attached venom sac should be carefully *scraped* (never squeezed, since this injects more venom) from the skin. If bitten by a black widow or brown recluse spider or a scorpion, the victim should lie down at once. A cold pack should be applied to the bite and medical assistance obtained immediately. The same applies to someone who is attacked by a swarm of biting or stinging insects. About 5 percent of Americans are allergic to insect stings: if weakness, headache, breathing difficulties, body rash, or stomach cramps occur, you may be one of the 5 percent. In these cases *immediate treatment is urgent.* Shock and even death can occur quickly. If you know you are allergic, your doctor can provide you with an antivenom kit and injections to lessen the allergy. You should take the antivenom kit with you to all games and practice sessions and notify your coach at the season's start that you have an insect-sting allergy.

**Blisters**   Small blisters should be covered with a small pad and adhesive dressing. Large blisters should be left intact and covered with a sterile bandage. Blisters can be a sign that something else is not right: shoes don't fit, glove isn't broken in, etc.

**Cramps**   Cramps are painful, sustained muscle contractions. When an exercising muscle doesn't get enough oxygen it may cramp. Stop using the muscle right away. Slowly and carefully stretch it out. Some people find that massage and heat are also helpful. (Taking time to warm up properly and stretch out completely right before you play can help prevent cramping during games and practice sessions.) Fluids, especially water, before and during games will decrease cramps, especially on hot and humid days.

**Cuts**   Superficial cuts should be cleaned with an antiseptic or iodine spray, and a dry dressing should be applied. Deeper cuts may require stitches. Sometimes long, thin strips of adhesive material can be applied under tension across a wound to hold it together. The cut is then covered with a sterile bandage.

**Dental Emergencies**   If you knock out or crack a tooth, go to your dentist immediately. Save the tooth and take it with you to the dentist. Perhaps it can be replaced in your mouth. If the tooth is just knocked loose or out of position, readjust it in its socket and hold it in place by biting on gauze, then visit your dentist as soon as possible to make sure there is no serious damage.

**Dislocations or Displacement of Bones** Sometimes the bones forming a joint can get dislocated or "out of joint." These dislocations may involve the shoulder, hip, finger, knee, or any other joint, and they are extremely painful. *Do not attempt to correct the dislocation yourself.* You could cause a great deal more damage. The victim must be transported to a hospital emergency room immediately, and with as little movement of the affected area as possible. Ice may be applied to the site, and it should be kept elevated to decrease swelling and pain.

**Broken Bones** If there is a broken bone or even the possibility of broken bone, take the injured person to a hospital emergency room as soon as possible. Do not move the injured part any more than is absolutely necessary. Apply ice and try to keep the injured part from moving by using a splint or a pillow. Do not give the person *anything* by mouth—food, drink, or medication. Sometimes broken bones can only be set properly when you have been put to sleep in the hospital. Your stomach should be completely empty for this procedure. Keep the person lying down and warm. If you think that the injury might involve the head, neck, or spine, keep the victim still and do not allow rocking motion. Call an ambulance right away. If the hand, arm, or collarbone is involved, a sling can be applied if it is not too painful. Just knot a loop of cloth behind the neck and rest the arm inside the draped portion. You can use a jacket or shirt or whatever else works.

**Strains and Sprains**  Strains refer to muscles and sprains refer to ligaments. Muscle fibers can be stretched and torn. A tear can be very tiny or fairly large. The kind of soreness you feel a few hours after a good practice or a tough game probably comes from stretching lots of the fibers in your muscles beyond their regular length. If you are in good condition and have done your warm-up and flexibility exercises before playing, you will probably have fewer muscle strains when play begins. If you aren't in very good shape or haven't warmed up or stretched enough, then you'll notice the soreness more. Muscle tears (or strains) can happen if the fibers are stretched beyond what they are used to. These tears need plenty of time to heal properly.

Ligaments are thick bands of tough tissue that connect bones together. You have ligaments at all of the joints in your arms and legs. Ligaments that are stretched beyond their normal limit can develop tears called sprains. If applied immediately, a cold pack or aerosol refrigerant will reduce pain and swelling. Keep the injured part elevated and as still as possible. After twenty minutes, replace the cold pack with a thick bandage (such as an elastic bandage) to provide support, but be careful not to make it so tight that it interferes with blood circulation. Remember that sometimes it's hard to tell the difference between a sprain and a broken bone: if there's any doubt, treat the injury like a broken bone.

**Eye Injuries**  For a black eye, apply an ice pack or cold compress immediately. The injury could be serious. If there is any bleeding or if swelling increases, get medical assistance. Apply a clean, sterile dressing. The injured person should lie flat. If an eyelash, piece of dust, insect, or other object gets into your eye, get your coach to help you locate the object. If it's on the inner surface of the lower lid, pull the lower lid down and lift off the object with the tip of a clean, moistened handkerchief or cotton swab. If it's on the upper lid, you should look down and grasp the upper lashes and pull the upper lid forward and down over the lower lid. If that doesn't work, try to pull the upper eyelid inside out and gently rub a cotton swab across the inside. With any luck, you'll be able to get whatever was bothering the eye onto the swab and remove it. Afterward, rinse the eye thoroughly with water for several minutes.

A team first-aid kit is a good idea. Its contents should include:

1. Sterile gauze and bandages (including gauze rolls in widths of one and three inches)

2. Antiseptic solution

3. Ace bandage wrap

4. Chemical cold pack

5. Scissors

6. Cotton swabs

7. Saline eye irrigation solution (Dacriose)

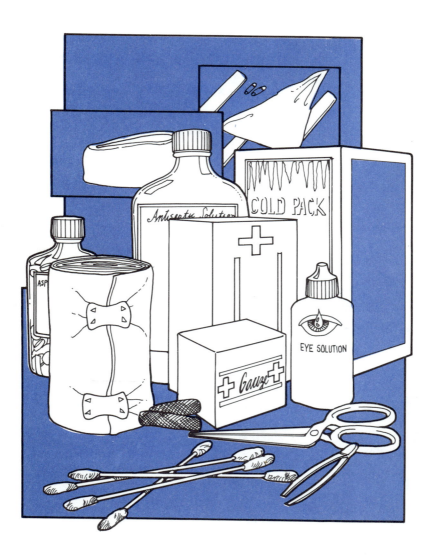

8. Tweezers

9. Triangular bandage and safety pins

10. Multipurpose splint or splints—the inflatable kind if you can afford them or else cardboard substitutes

11. Cervical (neck) collar

12. Aspirin and acetaminophen (such as Tylenol)

13. Ammonia inhaler (ampules)

# CHAPTER FIVE

# Eating Well

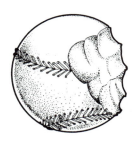

Have you heard the saying, "You are what you eat?" It's true. What you eat, drink, and breathe is what your body uses to build and repair your muscles, organs, blood, bones, teeth—every part of you. Food is also the raw material which your body turns into energy. You need energy to keep your body warm and to provide fuel for your working muscles. When you play baseball, you need extra energy.

Foods contain different kinds of nutrients—things that nourish, such as proteins (body builders), carbohydrates (a source of energy), fats (a reserve fuel), vitamins and minerals, and, most important of all, water. Eating right means enjoying a "balanced" system of eating; that is, enough of each of these nutrients every day. One way to balance all the nutrients is to follow the Basic Four Food Groups. Most foods can be placed into these four basic groups. When you eat the suggested amounts from each group every day, you'll be getting the nutrients you need to play your best.

# The Basic Four

1. Dairy or milk group (four glasses daily, or substitute cheese or ice cream for one glass).

2. Fruit and vegetable group (four or more servings). Aim for variety. Include an orange, grapefruit, or tomato (or juice) each day, along with a green or yellow vegetable.

3. Meat group (two servings), includes fish, chicken, eggs, dried beans, and nuts.

4. Bread and cereal group (four servings), includes whole-grain and enriched breads, cereals, pasta, and rice.

**Water** Remember to take plenty of liquids—water, milk, and juice—each day. Sometimes you hear about athletes losing weight or "making" weight by getting rid of fluids. They cut back on what they drink as well as trying to increase the amount they perspire. This is a dangerous way to shed pounds. Without the right amount of fluid in your body you just don't function well: your reactions are slower, your speed is slower, and your endurance is reduced. There should be a time during all games and certainly during all practice sessions to get a drink of water. *Doing without water when you are thirsty isn't a sign of discipline, it is bad training practice.* Water should be available at all times during games and practices.

# GET THE NUTRIENTS YOUR ACTIVE LIFESTYLE DEMANDS.

## MAXIMIZE YOUR ENERGY LEVEL

with **Centinela Hospital Sports Vitamins,** the exclusive formula developed by Centinela Hospital Medical Center, Official Hospital for the

- 1984 Olympics
- PGA Tour
- Los Angeles Lakers
- Los Angeles Kings
- Lewitsky Dance Company

## HELP PREVENT FATIGUE AND IRRITABILITY FROM VITAMIN DEFICIENCY.

Replace nutrients depleted by stress with **Centinela Hospital Stress Formula Vitamins,** a scientific breakthrough based on years of stress research.

## NO OTHER VITAMINS CAN OFFER SO MUCH.

**Centinela Hospital Sports and Stress Formulas** contain at least 100% of the U.S. RDA of most vitamins and minerals. They're potent, yet safe.

**Complete the reverse side of this card and get active today.**

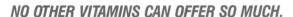

## MAIL THIS COUPON TODAY!

Centinela Hospital Medical Center, Pharmacy Department, 555 E. Hardy Street, P.O. Box 6015, Inglewood, CA 90312-6015

Centinela gives you the optimal levels of all vitamins that you need with each daily packet of 4 tablets and 1 capsule containing at least 100% of the U.S. RDA of most vitamins and minerals. It's virtually impossible for a single tablet to offer as much.

Choose one: ☐ Sports Formula    ☐ Stress Formula

Please send: ☐ One (1) box, 30 packets $15 (Ca. residents add $0.98 sales Tax)

☐ Three (3) boxes (save $4) $41 (Ca. residents add $2.67 sales Tax)

Add $2 shipping & handling

Order Total $ _____  $2.00

Charge to my: ☐ Visa    ☐ Mastercard    ☐ Check or money order enclosed
(make check payable to Centinela Hospital Medical Center)

Credit Card No. _____ Exp. date Mo./Yr. _____

Signature _____
(charge not valid unless signed)

Print Name _____

Address _____

City _____ State _____ Zip _____

Daytime Phone ( ___ ) _____
(In case we have a question about your order)

Send to: Centinela Hospital Medical Center, Pharmacy Department, 555 E. Hardy Street, P.O. Box 6015, Inglewood, CA 90312-6015

261

**Salt**   Many coaches and athletes are in the habit of taking salt tablets after a workout or game played on a warm day. This is probably not necessary. When you sweat, one of the ingredients of that perspiration is salt. Salt has two components, sodium and chloride. These elements, especially sodium, are necessary for body function. Your body has a very efficient internal regulation system for them. The diet of healthy Americans contains more than enough salt to meet their needs. In exercising, athletes lose lots of fluid, and in that fluid they lose some salt. But even exercising athletes have enough salt in a good, nutritious diet to replace all the salt that is lost during a workout or game. If you are getting low on sodium, your body will automatically take steps to raise the level by controlling the amount you lose in perspiration and urine.

**Carbohydrates**   In addition to eating a balanced diet, a young athlete should avoid eating too much sugar, fat, and salt. Instead, for best athletic performance, his or her diet should include foods with enough starch. Starch is really just one of several energy-providing substances called *carbohydrates*. Like starch, sugar is a carbohydrate and also is turned into energy. But sugary foods don't give anything else besides energy to the body. Foods like fruits and breads contain carbohydrates plus many other nutrients, such as vitamins, minerals, and fiber. Eating a candy bar provides only energy, and it provides energy only very briefly. After you eat the candy, the amount of sugar in your blood rises. Your body burns it for energy, then the blood sugar level drops. This rapid drop in blood sugar could rob you of important energy you need during a game—or any other time, for that matter. Foods with carbohydrates (fruits, vegetables) release their energy slowly, so your body doesn't experience that sharp drop in blood sugar level. Eating plenty of nutritious food cuts down your desire for sugary foods.

Foods with a lot of fat include butter, margarine and fried foods, like fried chicken or fried fish (the outer coating is the fatty part), french fries, and onion rings (again, it's the greasy coating). Foods with a lot of "cooked-in" fat include pastries, rich cakes and cookies, and meats like luncheon meats, hot dogs, and bacon. You shouldn't eat too many fatty foods because they fill you up and don't leave enough room for the good carbohydrates—starches—which are your best energy food.

Most kids don't have to think much about their weight. A few, however, are either overweight or underweight. What can you do to lose some extra pounds? You can:

1. Watch the size of your portions at meals. Take a regular-sized serving instead of heaping your plate full.

2. Cut back on sugary, fatty snacks like doughnuts, potato chips, candy bars and soft drinks.

3. Enjoy fruit or frozen yogurt for dessert instead of pie, cake, or ice cream.

4. Drink water instead of soda when you are thirsty; switch from whole milk to low-fat or skim milk.

Chocolate milk has lots of extra calories from sugar.

5. If you must order fried foods, get the regular and not the extra-crispy kind.

6. Make sure you get plenty of exercise.

What if you feel that gaining a few extra pounds would be a good idea? Try some of these suggestions:

1. Add a little extra to your plate at each meal. Have just a little more than your regular serving size.

2. Don't skip meals. Eat breakfast, lunch, and dinner.

3. Eat between meals. You can have fruit, granola bars, peanut butter and crackers, cheese, or yogurt.

4. Include many starches, such as potatoes, corn, and peas, in your meals. Whole-grain breads and cereals are good, too.

5. Ask for whole milk instead of low-fat milk.

**What to Eat Before the Game** An overly full stomach and "pregame jitters" could add up to stomach cramps when you need them least. To give your system time to finish digesting your pregame meal, try to eat about three hours before game time.

Before a game, avoid fatty foods, fried foods, cheese,

cream, butter, oil, and nuts because these take a long time to digest.

Select familiar favorites that do not upset your stomach. While some athletes can eat spicy or strongly flavored foods, such foods give others a bellyache during a game. Let common sense and what you have comfortably eaten in the past guide you.

Do drink plenty of liquids with your pregame meal, especially in hot weather. Supplying your body with enough water is an important step in getting ready to play your best for the whole game. Fruit juice (perhaps diluted with water) and bouillon are good choices. A glass of skim milk or low-fat milk could be included, too. Whole milk takes longer to leave your stomach.

Drink another glass of water one-and-a-half hours before game time. This allows enough time for the excess to go through your system and helps your body's "cooling system" through a sweaty game.

Instead of choosing a hefty helping of meat as the star of your pregame meal, choose a good supply of carbohydrates, like bread to build a sandwich, and fruit, vegetables and/or potatoes, rice, or pasta, prepared with very little (if any) added fat.

**A Word on "Junk Food"**   Are you a "junk-food junkie"? Eating junk food—quickie foods that have lots of sugar, fat, and salt and few other important nutrients—may not keep you from playing baseball. But take a break from your chips and doughnuts to think about this: If you had a Porsche, would you fuel it with cheap gas? It could run on cheap gas, but it couldn't win a race.

In much the same way, you might be able to get by on junk food, but you won't look, feel, or play your best if junk food crowds out other good foods.

## Sample Menus for Game Days

The suggested amounts will vary with the player's age, size, and activity level. Menus are offered only as suggestions, not to be rigidly followed.

On the day of an afternoon game, follow the basic outline given below.

### Breakfast (about 7 A.M.)

Fruit juice and/or fruit—½ cup or more

Cereal—¾ cup or more

Toast or English muffin—1 or 2 slices, very lightly buttered

Egg—1 or 2, or other protein food like *lean* meat or 2 tablespoons of peanut butter (avoid bacon and sausage, which are high in fat)

8 oz. of low-fat or skim milk

1 or 2 glasses of water, if desired

## Early Lunch (about 10:30–11 A.M.)

6–8 oz. of soup (not a creamed soup)

1 sandwich made with 1 to 2 oz. of *lean* meat (turkey or chicken are good choices)

Fruit and/or fruit juice

8 oz. of low-fat or skim milk

1–2 glasses of water, if desired

## Postgame Snack (optional)—to replenish fluids, minerals, and carbohydrates

Fruit juice or fruit

Light sandwich or crackers with cheese or peanut butter

## Dinner

Meat, fish or poultry—3 oz. or more

Potato, rice, or other starchy vegetable—½ cup or more

Vegetable and/or salad

Bread

Dessert of choice

8–12 oz. of milk

Additional water as desired

On the day of an evening game, follow the same basic outline, but morning and noon meals may be larger and dinner should be smaller, served at least three hours before game time with dessert saved to be eaten as a postgame snack.

# INDEX

# BIOGRAPHIES

Frank Wilson Jobe, M.D. is Associate Clinical Professor of Orthopaedics, University of Southern California School of Medicine; Emeritus member of the Board of Trustees of Centinela Hospital Medical Center, Co-Founder and Executive Medical Director of the National Athletic Health Institute and Medical Director, Biomechanics Laboratory, Centinela Hospital Medical Center. Dr. Jobe is the ortho-paedic consultant to the PGA TOUR. He is a Fellow of the American College of Surgeons and the American

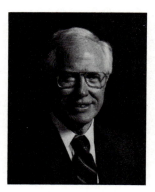

Academy of Orthopaedic Surgeons and chairman of its Committee on the Shoulder and Elbow. He is a founding member of the International Society of the Knee, the American Orthopaedic Society for Sports Medicine and the American Shoulder and Elbow Surgeons.

A consultant to the President's Council on Physical Fitness and Sports, Dr. Jobe is team physician to the Los Angeles Dodgers. He is the author of more than 40 medical articles and has given hundreds of lectures on orthopedic and sports injury subjects.

Diane Radovich Moynes, M.S., R.P.T. is Assistant Administrator in charge of Research at Centinela Hospital Medical Center. Formerly the Director of the Biomechanics Laboratory, Ms. Moynes is a registered physical therapist and a clinical specialist in neurology. She has lectured at USC in neuroanatomy, biostatistics, and physical therapy. She has published fifteen professional papers and given numerous presentations at conferences and meetings.

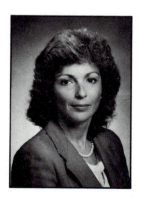

# LOWER YOUR GOLF SC⬤RE

with **30 EXERCISES FOR BETTER GOLF**, the world's first scientific exercise program designed specifically for golfers.

**With 30 EXERCISES FOR BETTER GOLF, you can:**
- Increase muscle strength and flexibility
- Drive the ball further
- Make better contact
- Build endurance
- Play more consistently
- Decrease risk of injury

**Professionals on the PGA Tour use 30 EXERCISES FOR BETTER GOLF. They report:**
- Less soreness
- Increased flexibility
- Better, harder practice sessions
- More accurate swings
- An incredible competitive edge.

**Perfect for golfers at all levels.**
Develop the program that works best for you and your game, regardless of age or ability level. Start slowly and work at your own pace and watch your golf score go down.

**Developed by sports experts.**
These exercises were designed by Centinela Hospital Medical Center, the Official Hospital for the PGA Tour.

**Give 30 EXERCISES FOR BETTER GOLF** to the golfer you love.

**Complete the reverse side of this card and start improving your game today.**

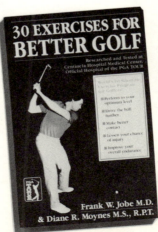

30 EXERCISES FOR BETTER GOLF

Researched and Tested at Centinela Hospital Medical Center, Official Hospital of the PGA TOUR

World's first Scientific Exercise Program for Golfers!
- Perform at your optimum level
- Drive the ball further.
- Make better contact
- Lessen your chance of injury
- Improve your overall endurance

Frank W. Jobe M.D. & Diane R. Moynes M.S., R.P.T.

TEAR HERE

# MAIL THIS COUPON TODAY!

Please send me _____ copies of **30 EXERCISES FOR BETTER GOLF** @ $7.95 each plus $1.55 for postage and handling —

☐ $9.50 total per book (non-Calif. residents) or

☐ $10.00 total per book (Calif. residents — sales tax per book)

☐ My check or money order for $ _____ is enclosed, payable to Champion Press.

Please charge my VISA _____ MASTERCARD _____ Expiration Date _____

Credit card number: _____ - _____ - _____ - _____

Signature: _____

(charge not valid unless signed)

Print Name: _____

Street Address: _____

City: _____ State: _____ Zip: _____

Send to: Champion Press, P.O. Box 7000-166, Palos Verdes Peninsula, CA 90274